Healthy Smile, Healthy Body!

Your Mouth is the Gateway to Health.

By

Gregory LaMorte, DDS

To my parents who gave me the gift of education

To my family, especially Pat, who loves me even when

I do not deserve it

Table of Contents

Preface

Dealing with dental issues is not usually on top of anyone's list of favorite things. Bad past experiences, lack of knowledge and believing in dental myths can keep you from making your smile a priority.

The information that I am sharing in this book is designed to help you make an informed decision about some of the forms of treatment to restore your oral health, and discuss ways to care for your teeth. It addresses five critical topics that impact immediate concerns of oral health as well as total body health; oral hygiene, gum diseases, treatment, dental implants, and receding gums.

Dental care is very personal. It is important to ask pertinent questions about recommended treatment and additional options. It is our hope that this book will make you a better patient by helping you become a more informed patient.

A healthy mouth has great value. In fact, preventive care is one of the best investments you can make. You can be sure that treatment now will give greater value and cost less, probably, then treatment in the future.

The first thing most people take notice of is your smile. Having missing teeth or other obvious aesthetic problems could adversely affect one's social or professional life.

Dr. Gregory LaMorte, a practicing Periodontist for over 20 years, shares his knowledge about current procedures in periodontics, dental implant and some cosmetic dental procedures. As a skilled dentist in over fourteen treatments and procedures, Dr. LaMorte has the skill to perform complex procedures, yet he also has the ability to explain the procedures in words of one syllable! He has taught courses on many different subjects related to periodontics, implant dentistry and 3D imaging. He has served on the American Dental Association Council on Annual Sessions, and he has served on the Board of Trustees of the New Jersey Dental Association. He serves as the 2015-2016 President of the New Jersey Dental Association.

SECTION I

What is a Healthy Mouth?

Dr. Thomas Fuller said, "Health is not valued until sickness comes" [1] Did you know that a healthy mouth promotes a healthy body? Regular dental visits do more than keep your smile pretty; they also can tell your dentist a lot about your overall health. Research suggests that the health of your mouth mirrors other conditions in your body.

According to the American Dental Association, [2] there is a relationship between gum disease and health complications such a heart disease. Women with gum disease also have a greater chance of having a low weight baby.[3] Other research shows that certain systemic diseases have signs or symptoms that can show up in the mouth including swollen gums, mouth ulcers, dry mouth, and gum problems.

Understanding the connection between a healthy mouth and good overall health not only will increase the quality of a person's healthy lifestyle, but may also act as a way to prevent future illnesses. Recognizing factors that impact oral hygiene is the easiest way to address challenges before they become chronic problems.

Additionally, when an acute situation occurs, this knowledge can allow a person to choose their best treatment choice.

The following chapters discuss how oral health can impact our overall health. They explain the connection between oral hygiene and disease or the absence of health. The chapters help you develop an understanding of the impact of oral hygiene, the warning signs, and risks that lead to gum disease and we briefly describe certain treatments that have proven successful.

Chapter 1: Oral Hygiene

Chapter 1: **Oral Hygiene**

What are the diseases connected to oral hygiene?

Diabetes, leukemia, oral cancer, heart disease and kidney disease can present in the mouth or have a connection to oral hygiene. Poor hygiene and avoiding regular dental cleanings can lead to oral and facial pain, heart disease, and digestive problems. Digestion begins with the chemical processes in your mouth. Problems in the mouth can lead to stomach or other digestive disorders. Lack of teeth or teeth in poor condition can make chewing difficult, leading to digestive problems.

Additionally, without front teeth, you will have difficulty biting into things. Dentists call it incising. Loss of front teeth makes it difficult or impossible to bite into a sandwich or a piece of fruit. Without back teeth, we call them molars, it is difficult to grind food into pieces small enough to be swallowed and digested properly.

What is the result of poor oral hygiene?

The number one problem in adults that leads to tooth loss is gum disease or periodontal disease. It was previously known as pyorrhea. Now we say periodontitis. Periodontitis causes the gums to separate from the teeth and leads to bone loss around the teeth. The bone supports the tooth and gives the tooth strength, just like cement gives strength to a building's foundation. Without enough bone to support the tooth, the tooth becomes weak and sometimes loose. Chewing becomes more difficult. If left untreated, the bone loss could lead to tooth loss.

What are the warning signs of poor dental hygiene?

Warning signs include gums that bleed, are red, swollen or tender, gums that have separated or pulled away from your teeth, receding gums, painful chewing, persistent bad breath or a bad taste in your mouth. Teeth that are loose or separating, a change in the way your teeth fit together, or any change in the fit of a dental appliance are also warning signs that you should not ignore. All of these symptoms tell you something is wrong. Addressing them as soon as you become aware of them will allow for quicker healing and have less of a financial impact on the treatment.

What are the risks of developing gum disease?

The risks include poor oral hygiene, crooked teeth that are hard to keep clean, smoking or chewing tobacco, stress, immuno-deficiencies, defective fillings, bridges that no longer fit, as well as some genetic factors. Hormonal changes including pregnancy and oral contraceptives can be a factor. Medications can cause side effects that cause gum issues including steroids, certain drugs for seizures, certain cancer drugs and drugs that cause dry mouth. Some drugs for heart disease and blood pressure called calcium channel blockers cause thickening of the gums called hyperplasia. If you suspect there is gum disease, then you should see a dentist, or if you prefer a dental specialist, call a periodontist.

The primary risk factor is the plaque that forms on our teeth, but other factors can affect your gums as well. Age can be a factor on the basis that the longer you keep your teeth; the more likely it is that you could develop gum disease. The Center for Disease Control indicates that over 70% of adults over 65 have some evidence of periodontitis.[4] Smoking is associated with other diseases like cancer, lung disease, and heart disease. Tobacco users are at increased risk of periodontal disease because the direct effect of the smoke on the gums. Periodontists say that smoking kills teeth.

Genetics can also be a factor; you don't inherit periodontal disease, but what you do inherit is a susceptibility or tendency toward it. It is often recommended that adults with periodontal disease have their children examined, especially adult children, so that if they show signs of early gum disease it can be dealt with through early intervention and prevent the disease from progressing.

Stress is also a factor; it's linked to hypertension and other health problems. It's a risk factor for gum disease because it makes it more difficult for the body to fight off infections. And as stated, Periodontitis is a chronic illness. Medications, such as oral contraceptives, which are hormones, antidepressants, and certain heart medications can affect your oral health. Drugs for high blood pressure cause the most widely seen effects on oral hygiene because of the chemicals called calcium channel blockers.

Years ago we used to see a lot of problems associated with anti-epilepsy drugs, but the drugs that caused the gum problems are rarely used anymore. That's why it is important to share your health information with your dentist.

Clenching and grinding your teeth can also put extra force on the bones that surround your teeth. Usually, one of two things happens in people who clench or grind their teeth; we call grinding bruxism. Either they wear their teeth down, which is not good because it can lead to tooth sensitivity, or if the teeth don't wear down from the grinding, the transmitted force to the gum, bone and teeth can cause the teeth to become loose. If you discover that you are clenching or grinding you should report it to your dentist or your periodontist.

Finally, other systemic conditions affect or interfere with the body's inflammatory system and can worsen the condition of your gums. Specifically, diabetes and autoimmune diseases cause the body to turn on itself such as rheumatoid arthritis, lichen planus, and lupus, and these often manifest themselves first in your mouth.

Chapter 2: Gum Disease

Chapter 2: **Gum Disease**

What causes gum disease?

Plaque causes gum disease; it's the sticky film of germs that continually form on our teeth. It may lead to a chronic infection of the tissue that surrounds the tooth and bone that lead to tooth loss in adults. The way to prevent that type of gum disease is with regular dental visits that include cleanings and exams that periodontists call probing along with good home care that involves brushing and flossing daily. Unfortunately, gum disease is often painless so that you don't know that you have it, and that's why it is important to see your dentist regularly for dental cleanings and evaluations.

What are the connections between gum disease and other health issues?

Research between systemic disease and periodontal disease is ongoing. The risks in non-conclusive studies indicate an association between severe gum disease with several other health conditions, such as diabetes or heart disease. Unfortunately, it is also possible to have gum disease and no warning signs. This most commonly happens in smokers because smoking causes the blood vessels in the gum to close down so bleeding on brushing doesn't occur.

That's why it is important to see a dentist regularly and have the periodontal exams to check for problems that can't be seen just by looking. Also, good self-care at home is essential not only to prevent periodontal disease, but after treatment, it helps to prevent periodontal disease from recurring.

The important thing to know is that gum disease is preventable. You don't have to lose your teeth. What you need to do is brush your teeth twice a day, clean between your teeth daily with dental floss. Your toothbrush doesn't reach far enough between your teeth. Eat a balanced diet and schedule regular dental visits to keep your teeth for a lifetime.

How does gum disease affect women?

A variety of factors may impact a woman's periodontal health. During puberty, an increased level of hormones causes increased blood circulation in the gums. Puberty may cause increase gum sensitivity, and lead to a greater reaction from irritation including foods and plaque. During this time, the gums may get swollen, turn red, and feel tender. Also, during menstruation, some women occasionally develop gingivitis. A woman with this condition may develop bleeding gums, bright red or swollen gums, or sores in their mouth.

Menstrual gingivitis typically begins right before a woman's period and clears up once her period has started. Some studies have suggested the possibility of an additional risk factor during pregnancy from periodontal disease. Pregnant women who have periodontal disease may be more likely to have a baby born pre-term or with low birth weight. However, more research is needed to confirm how periodontal disease may affect pregnancy outcomes. Remember, all infections are a cause for concern among pregnant women because they pose a risk to the baby. The American Academy of Periodontology recommends that woman considering pregnancy have a periodontal evaluation and frequent cleanings while pregnant. [5]

Women who are menopausal or post-menopausal also may experience changes in their mouth. They may get discomfort including dry mouth, burning sensations, and altered taste. Also, menopausal gingivostomatitis affects a small percentage of women. Gums that look dry or shiny, bleed easily, and range from pale to dark red mark this condition. Most women find that estrogen supplements help to relieve these symptoms.

How does gum disease affect men?

Research shows that periodontal disease is higher in men. It occurs in about 55% of men and only in about 38% of women.[6] Why does this happen? We think it is because men are less likely to go to the dentist unless they have pain or because men have worse indicators of periodontal health than women.

There is a higher incidence of plaque, tartar, which is hardened plaque, and bleeding on probing. However, periodontal health in men is critical because it could affect other health conditions. Men who have problems with prostate have an increased antigen called Prostate Specific Antigen (PSA). We know that men who have inflamed, infected, or have cancer of the prostate have increased PSA levels. Research shows that men who have a periodontal disease can also have an increased PSA level than men without periodontal problems.[7] Therefore, there is a connection between the health of the prostate and dental and periodontal health and visa-verse, but there needs to be more research.

Recent research does indicate that periodontal disease and cardiovascular disease are associated.[8] Having periodontal disease may increase your risk of cardiovascular disease. Both diseases are chronic inflammation. Researchers believe that inflammation is the connection between the two conditions.[9] Since men are more likely to develop heart disease than women, maintaining periodontal health is another way to reduce the risk.

What is Gingivitis?

The early stage of gum disease is called gingivitis. If you have gingivitis, your gums may look red or swollen and at that stage it is reversible because it is early. Usually it can be eliminated by a professional cleaning at a dental office followed by daily brushing and flossing. If left uncontrolled, it may lead to the more advanced disease. We described gums separating and leading to bone loss. Remember, that condition is called periodontitis, as we noted previously. Read on for a full definition of periodontitis.

What is Periodontitis?

In periodontitis, the plaque can spread below the gum line, and it starts to loosen the attachment of the gum to the tooth. What occurs is that germs in plaque produce toxins. They irritate the gum, and those toxins stimulate your body to act against itself. The chronic inflammation causes the gum to separate from the tooth more and destroys the attachment. When the gum separates from the tooth, they form pockets. Pockets are spaces between the gum and the teeth, and those pockets can become infected. As the disease progresses, the pockets deepen and destroys more gum tissue and bone.

This process has very mild and sometimes no symptoms. Eventually, if left untreated, the teeth can become loose and may have to be removed. Dentists have identified a few forms of Periodontitis; chronic, aggressive, and necrotizing.

Chronic Periodontitis

Chronic periodontitis happens when you have inflammation in the supporting tissue around the teeth, the gum, and the bone. And leads to progressive loss of gum attachment and progressive bone loss and this is the most frequent form of periodontitis. It is characterized by the pockets, as mentioned before, and involves gum deterioration. It is the most common in adults but can occur at any age, and it usually proceeds very slowly.

Chronic periodontitis affects over 40% of the adults over 30 in the United States and it leads to tooth loss.[10] If left untreated it slowly progresses over time and eventually the teeth loosen and start moving. The most common form of peritonitis can occur at any age, but it usually occurs in adults. It can get worse slowly, but there can be periods of rapid progression.

Aggressive Periodontitis

Aggressive periodontitis happens in patients who are otherwise healthy, and it involves rapid detachment and bone loss and usually happens within families. If a family member receives a diagnosed of aggressive periodontitis, siblings should be checked also and make sure they don't exhibit aggressive peritonitis.

Aggressive periodontitis, previously referred to as juvenile periodontitis, is a very fast moving and highly destructive form of periodontal disease that can occur in even healthy patients.

Commonly what happens is there is a rapid loss of gum or bone around teeth in only certain areas of the mouth.

Necrotizing Periodontitis

Necrotizing periodontal disease is an infection characterized by the top layer of the gum separating from the underlying connective tissue, leaving sore red gums. It occurs most commonly in people with systemic diseases such as HIV, malnutrition, or patients who are immunosuppressed. But it can also occur in stressful situations. This type of periodontal disease often requires treatment that includes the use of antibiotics.

What can you do about gum disease?

First, you need to improve your oral hygiene routine at home. Oral hygiene includes brushing, flossing, and rinsing on a daily basis. Second, you need to see your dentist regularly to help keep your mouth in top shape and allow your dentist to watch for developments that may signal other health issues. A dental exam can also detect inadequate home care, growth problems, and improper jaw alignments.

SECTION II

What are the Best Interventions?

Medical treatments, referred to as procedures or interventions, are usually performed to help treat or cure a condition. The most important thing to understand about dental treatments is there is no cookie cutter approach. A lot depends on specific cases and the expertise of the dentist performing the treatment. A dentist may have the expertise to do specific procedures and lack the expertise to do other procedures depending on where they went to school and what additional training they have received.

Also, periodontal disease is not cured in the sense that you can cure a cold and a sore throat, but rather a dentist performs a treatment. If you inherited a tendency to periodontal disease or have had treatment for periodontal disease, you need to stay on a maintenance program of continuing care which is basically one visit cleanings and probing in order to prevent your gum disease from recurring.

Dentistry is not just science, but art. Two dentist's opinion can differ on how the exact problem can be handled. Therefore, the general advice is that any questions should be addressed to your periodontist, and they can answer specific questions about your particular condition.

The next two chapters discuss two types of interventions; first those applied to existing teeth, such as scaling and root planing, pocket reduction, laser treatments, grafting, and tray delivery systems and, secondly, those involved in replacing the tooth root with a titanium post (a dental implant).

Chapter 3: **Treatment**

Chapter 3: **Treatment**

Who should treat periodontal disease?

So, you suspect you have gum disease, and decide to see a periodontist, what should you do? You could consult the site of the American Academy of Periodontology which is www.perio.org for a periodontist in your area and then call to schedule an exam.

Instead of leaving your dental treatment to one dental professional, you should consider having your dentist work with a periodontist, who is also actively involved in the treatment of your periodontal disease. We call this the team approach. The team approach helps your regular dentist who is familiar with your dental and medical history and your periodontist who has extensive training in treating periodontal, collaborate and come up with a treatment plan that works best in your individual case.

Treatment is not from a cookbook; each patient needs an individualized plan. Not every patient needs the same treatment, nor would they benefit from the same treatment. Someone needs to determine, in your particular case, what is the best form of treatment, as well as the extent of treatment. This determination occurs with a thorough examination and x-rays during the first appointment.

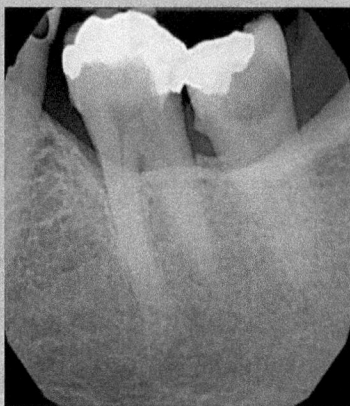

This sixty-nine year old female patient came to see me for a second opinion on treatment that had been recommended to her. It included clinical crown lengthening, root canal therapy and repairing the tooth with a post, core and crown for tooth #17.

When I examined her mouth, I notice that opposite the teeth in Figure 1 there was a tooth missing.

The first thing this nice lady needed was options.

These are the options in no particular order:

Clinical crown lengthening, root canal therapy and repairing the tooth with a post, core and crown
Extraction of tooth #17 and replacement of tooth #3
Extraction of tooth #17 and no replacements

What would you do?

She decided to extract tooth #17 and has not decided about the opposite tooth.

What happens at the first appointment?

At the first appointment, the periodontist will take measurements of the crevices around every tooth in your mouth, chart the missing teeth and take x-rays to check the bone around your teeth. Based on the findings, the periodontist will discuss treatment options with you. People often ask if the treatment will hurt. If it's done carefully by someone with a lot of experience, it is rarely very painful.

The exam consists of using a thin instrument that has depth markings to determine the depth of pockets around every tooth in the mouth. Because, as I said before, gum disease can be localized around one tooth or could be generalized around all teeth. We also use x-rays. X-rays are important because they allow us to see where we can't see by looking, basically a way to look inside and see the condition of the bone around each tooth.

Many dentists have the ability to take what's called a cone beam x-ray, which is a three-dimensional x-ray that determines how much bone is missing. Standard x-rays that dentists take are two-dimensional, like a picture. They show height and width, but don't show depth. However, the three-dimensional picture shows us exactly how it looks; showing us the tooth and the bone in three dimensions.

Keep in mind, that to have a proper diagnosis you need to have a periodontal probe that checks the depth of the narrow crevice around each tooth, and you need to have x-rays to look at the bone around each tooth.

How much will the treatment cost?

Once there is a determination that treatment is necessary and what type of treatment will be best, then the periodontist should discuss with you how much the treatment will cost, what the expected results are, and how you could keep your gums healthy going forward. The cost of the initial exam varies from area to area but in the New York metropolitan area, it can cost upwards of $200.

What type of treatments does a periodontist do?

As a dental expert in treating periodontal disease, periodontists receive upwards of three years of specialized training in both gum surgery and non-surgical treatment of gum disease and gum issues. They are also experts in replacing missing teeth with implants. Non-surgical treatment could include scaling and root planing, which is careful cleaning of the root surface to remove plaque and tartar. In addition to scaling and root planing, periodontists often use adjunctive therapy such as antibiotics, or a local delivery of microbial agents. But the need for that is decided on a case by case basis.

Most periodontists agree that after scaling and root planning, some patients do not require additional treatment. The way to determine that is to return in the near future for an exam to have the probing done again. The periodontist will then use those numbers to determine how much your condition has improved due to the scaling and root planning. Even if no other treatment is necessary, you should continue with an ongoing maintenance therapy, usually every three months, to maintain your periodontal health. Did you know that most dentists, like me, have their teeth cleaned every three months?

Scaling and root planing

The purpose of scaling and root planing is to get the gum to reattach snugly around your teeth like a turtleneck shirt around your neck. When you have periodontal disease, the gum loosens and becomes detached from the tooth. Scaling and root planning, by cleaning the root of the tooth and smoothing it, allows the gum to reattach and for many pockets to get smaller. We clean the calculus deposits from the roots of the teeth from the deep periodontal pockets and also at the same time we smooth the roots to remove the bacterial toxins.

What happens if after the scaling and root planing the pocket still remains?

If the pockets are left untreated, at that point over time, they could become deeper and develop larger spaces for bacteria to live. That leads to other problems. When the pockets get deeper, the plaque hardens and becomes difficult and sometimes impossible for you to remove during routine home care. Also, as the bacteria get deeper into the gum, it becomes more aggressive. While it may cause fewer problems with the gum itself, the germs tend to cause more problems with the bone around your teeth because the environment changes. That's why the measurement of your pocket depth is so important. Having pockets relatively shallow are easier not only for your periodontist or dental hygienist to clean, but also shallow pockets are easier for you to maintain.

What is pocket reduction?

The dentist numbs the gum with a strong local anesthetic, such as Novocain. However, most of us now use Lidocaine or something called Septocaine. Once the gum is numb, we fold back the gum and remove disease-causing bacteria and deposits that we see on the root of the tooth. We also remove any diseased gum that remains attached to the area where the bone and gum meets the tooth.

Any irregular surfaces of the bone are smoothed to limit the area where the bacteria can hide and allow the gum tissue to better reattach. Toward the end of the procedure, we set the gum down closer to the bone to make the pocket smaller. This often leaves more of the tooth exposed above the gum line. Periodontists often say that it is better to have a longer tooth than a tooth no longer. And as we have already mentioned, reducing the pocket depth and eliminating existing bacteria tends to prevent additional damage and progression of the periodontal disease.

Sometimes scaling and root planing alone aren't enough, and the problem is that deeper pockets are harder to clean, even with scaling and root planning. Often, at a depth of more than five millimeters, bacteria and plaque can be left behind, so that's why sometimes the periodontist recommends pocket reduction treatment.

We also now have procedures that can regenerate some bone around the tooth to reverse some of the damage, but the indications are very specific and are best determined by a periodontist. Usually, we recommend regenerative procedures when the bone has been destroyed in a localized area, and we think that reversing the bone loss is possible. Typically, this can only be done in certain areas that meet specific criteria, but the basic procedure is the same. The periodontist peels back the gum and removes the disease-causing bacteria and deposits off the tooth root. We use materials or medicines to guide and encourage your body's natural ability to regenerate its own bone. Think of it as raising the bone instead of lowering the gum closer to the bone. These procedures, by minimizing the pocket, most likely will reduce the chance of the periodontal disease continuing and will make it easier for you and your periodontist to keep that area clean.

What is Laser Treatment?

Patients often ask about laser treatment of gum disease. The issue here is that each laser beam has a different wavelength and different lasers are used for different procedures. So, if your periodontist recommends the use of lasers, you should ask him specifically what he intends to use the laser for. Often the laser is just a mere substitute for a scalpel or cutting the gum, and other lasers are used to do certain regenerative procedures. That discussion is vital to have between you and your periodontist to determine the intended benefit of the treatment that is recommended.

What Additional Treatments Do Periodontists Perform?

Additional treatments involve gum graft surgery to cover exposed roots from damage to a gum or trauma to a gum. That is called gingival grafting. It can be done by moving oral tissue, usually from the roof of the mouth to replace lost gum over a tooth. This is called an autogenous graft. A similar procedure can also be done with donor tissue. Ask about your options and know which procedure has been recommended to you. Each procedure has its advantages and disadvantages.

We do other procedures to repair a broken or decayed tooth. One procedure is called dental crown lengthening. We remove gum tissue, and sometimes bone, around a tooth to expose more of the natural tooth so a repair is possible. We often do it to allow proper capping of a tooth.

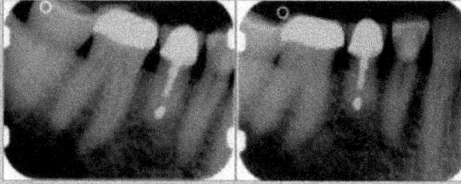

This is a sixty year old man who had been under my care to treat an autoimmune condition, lichen planus. At one visit he told me that his dentist found a problem with tooth #29. It is the tooth in the center of the right x-ray.

The dentist told me that the post, core and crown came out and there was decay inside the tooth. The patient had the following options:

Extraction and a fixed bridge supported by teeth on either side of the space.

Extraction and graft followed later by an implant. (Delayed placement)

Extraction and immediate placement of an implant. (Immediate placement)

If you look at the flow sheets that refer to implants, you will see that the fastest treatment plan is to extract and immediately place an implant. Immediate placement saves the time that it would take for the socket to heal if we delayed implant placement.

On the other hand, there needs to be care in placing the implant. Without care and experience, it may lead to gum recession and the neck of the implant showing. The neck of the implant showing can effect the attractiveness of the final cap. In the back of the mouth that is not a real problem. In the front of the mouth, a person with a big smile can show the neck the implant and that is a problem.

The periodontist performs a very similar procedure on one tooth or several teeth to treat a problem called arrested passive eruption. Think of arrested passive eruption as a tooth or teeth having too much gum.

Tray delivery systems use a custom fit tray from the impression of your teeth, and then a patient uses the tray at home to deliver medications that have been prescribed by a dentist. The Food and Drug Administration (FDA) cleared the tray delivery systems since they are similar to fluoride trays used to prevent decay. However, the FDA clearance process did not determine which particular medication delivered via tray is the most effective or safe to treat gum disease. Due to limited testing, some consider this experimental or unproven.[11]

Chapter 4: **Dental Implants**

Chapter 4: **Dental Implants**

What makes the implant successful?

A dental implant involves replacing a tooth root with a titanium post. The posts come in several sizes, lengths, and diameters with different types of connections. There are different ways to connect a cap to a dental implant in order to replace a tooth or several teeth. Dental implants are 90% successful, in other words, there is seldom a problem with more than one out of 10.[12]

One reason for the success of implants is that the posts are titanium and unlike other metals, such as, stainless steel, bones bond directly to the titanium. If there was any other metal involved, the body would put fibers between the metal and the bone, and there would be movement or mobility which doesn't exist with a properly healed dental implant.

What are the steps in a full mouth replacement?

If someone needs a whole jaw full of teeth replaced, it can be done in several ways. One way is basically to make an entire jaw full of teeth supported by four implants. Different practitioners describe it in different ways. What happens is two implants in the front are placed parallel to each other, and two are placed toward the back of the mouth on an angle.

This approach is not a modality that I do. The reason I don't like it is because there is no redundancy. If you do six implants to replace a jaw full of teeth and one of those implants is not successful often five implants can be enough to support the teeth. However, rarely are three implants going to be sufficient to support a whole jaw full of teeth, especially if it is one of the implants in the back of the mouth. An entire section of that bridge could be lost because there is nothing at the end of that bridge holding it up.

What are the options to replace a missing tooth?

There are options! One is a fixed bridge. You can get a bridge when there are teeth on either side of the space. Teeth on either side of the gap are capped, a dummy tooth is attached to the caps and the caps are cemented onto the teeth. People call it a permanent bridge. A dentist doesn't use that term, because when you treat human beings what could be considered permanent? A dentist calls it a fixed bridge.

A second option is a removable bridge. The dentist makes a mold of the remaining teeth in the mouth. A dental laboratory makes a "partial" that clips onto some of the remaining teeth to hold it in place. The patient can snap it in and out as desired.

The third choice is an implant, where a post is put in the jaw and then a cap is fixed on to the post.

How Long Does the Implant Procedure Take?

We have included some of the flow charts (Figures 1, 2, 3) that show the timeline of the treatment processes. This gives our patients a visual explanation of the different possibilities of how the dentist performs the implant. With the ability to take 3-dimentional pictures, which are called a cone beam scans or a CBCT, the procedure of placing a single implant takes twenty five to thirty five minutes.

Timing – Option One

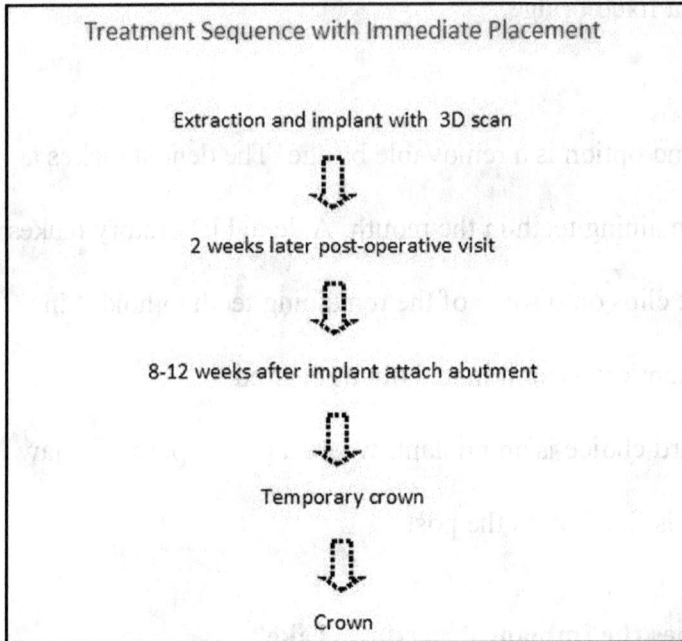

Treatment Sequence with Immediate Placement

Extraction and implant with 3D scan

⬇

2 weeks later post-operative visit

⬇

8-12 weeks after implant attach abutment

⬇

Temporary crown

⬇

Crown

Figure 1 – Treatment Sequence with Immediate Placement

Timing – Option Two

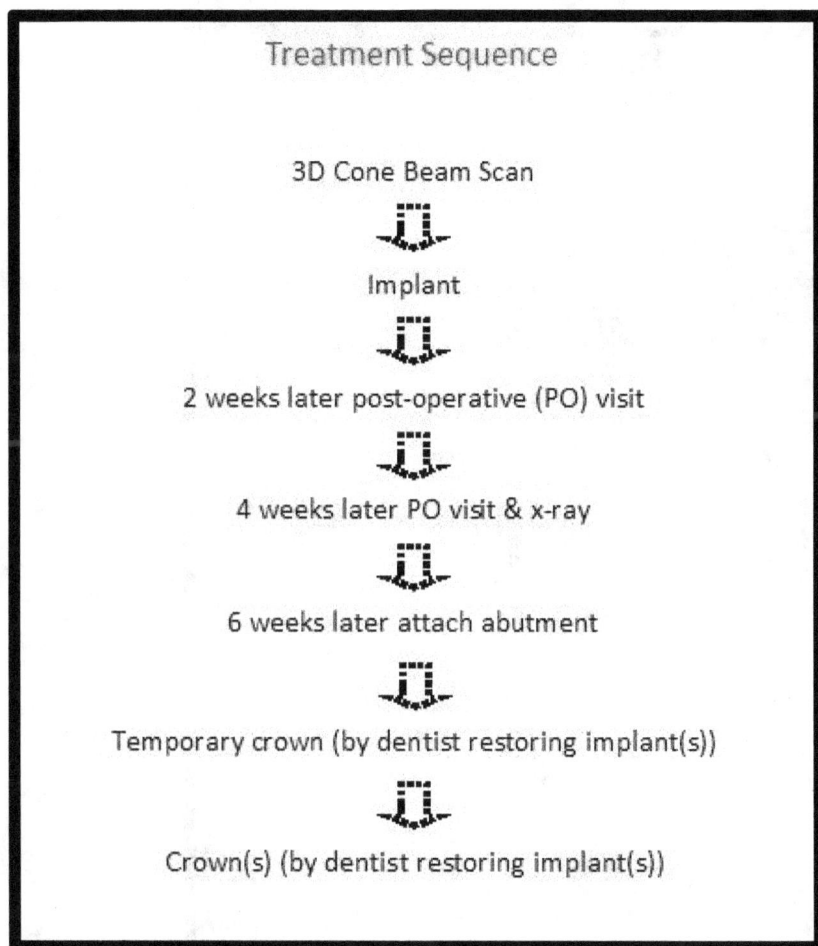

Treatment Sequence

3D Cone Beam Scan

Implant

2 weeks later post-operative (PO) visit

4 weeks later PO visit & x-ray

6 weeks later attach abutment

Temporary crown (by dentist restoring implant(s))

Crown(s) (by dentist restoring implant(s))

Figure 2 - Treatment Sequence for an implant placed a well healed site.

Timing – Option Three

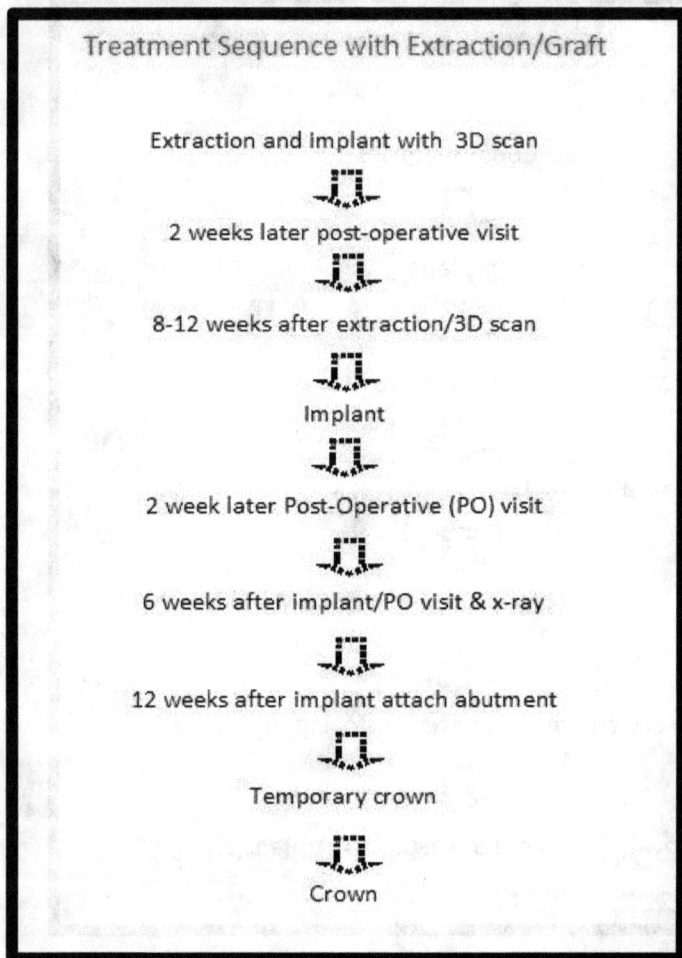

Treatment Sequence with Extraction/Graft

Extraction and implant with 3D scan

2 weeks later post-operative visit

8-12 weeks after extraction/3D scan

Implant

2 week later Post-Operative (PO) visit

6 weeks after implant/PO visit & x-ray

12 weeks after implant attach abutment

Temporary crown

Crown

Figure 3 – Treatment Sequence with Extraction/Graft followed later by an implant

What is involved in completing an implant?

Sometimes it is possible to extract a tooth and insert the implant in the same visit. This procedure is called an immediate placement. (Figure 1) In another approach, called a delayed placement, the dentist extracted the tooth at some point in the past, the site was allowed to heal, and then the dentist inserts the implant. (Figure 2) There is also something that is called immediate loading. The dentist surgically inserts the implant and the tooth is put on in the same visit.

The difficulty in an implant procedure is that it is impossible to predict the quality of healing in advance. Healing takes time. The dentist inserts the implant, waits, and evaluates the healing. Once healing has occurred, we make impressions for the cap.

Looking at the flow sheets, you will see that it takes several visits. The first visit is usually the exam, x-rays and the discussion of the recommended treatment plan. The second visit is placing the implants. The third visit is two weeks after to make sure the healing is going as uneventfully as possible and that there are no apparent complications. A month later we take an x-ray to look at the bone to see if the bone is healing against the implant, and we usually wait up

to twelve weeks to make impressions and a temporary cap.

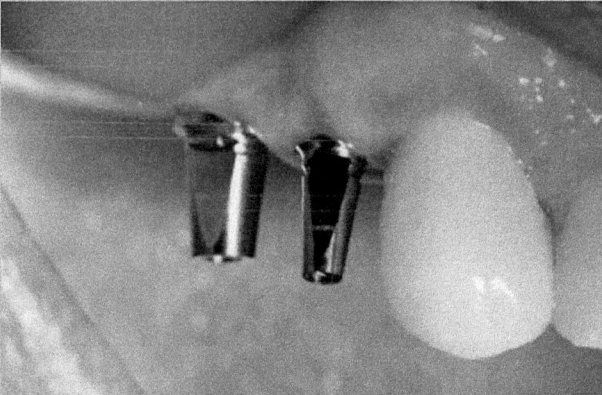

How a Titanium Post Works

This picture shows what a post (also called an abutment) looks like. They have a flat side, intended to prevent the tooth cap from spinning on the abutments.

Does the procedure hurt?

With proper local anesthesia such as lidocaine, or articaine, there is rarely pain during the procedure.

Do dentists give guarantees on the procedure?

Most dentists, not all, will replace the implant if it fails to integrate during the healing phase. It is a challenge to determine why it failed, if a lot of time has lapsed. You don't know what kind of care the patient has had. Did they do good home care? Do they have any habits like clenching or grinding? Every case needs to be carefully evaluated.

How long can an implant last?

With proper care, an implant may last a lifetime, but without proper care, it can develop gum disease just like a tooth can. Proper care for each individual patient must be personalized. Discuss this with your dentist. Most periodontists are ready, willing, and more than able to help with continuing care or maintenance care of those implants.

Team Approach

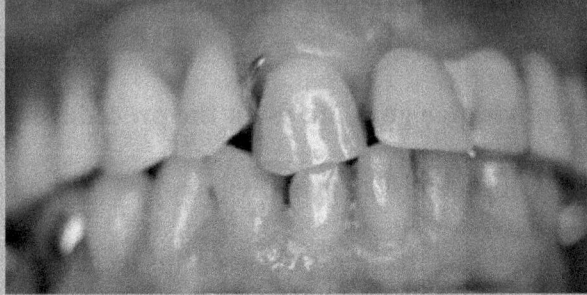

Fig. 1 Before

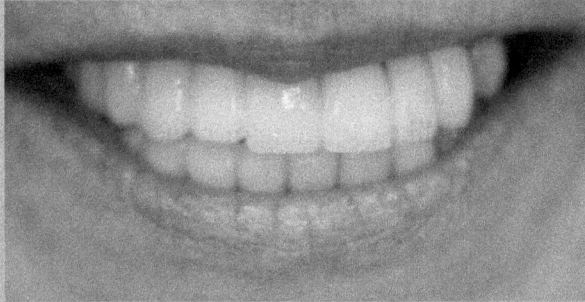

Fig. 2 After

The two pictures are the before and after of the same patient. She had been avoiding the dentist, but no longer wanted to tolerate her upper removable partial that attached with the silver clasp on her front tooth.

This was a team approach. Under sedation, I placed four dental implants in the upper right. Later I placed two implants in the lower left. These implants and her remaining teeth were later restored by Jeffrey Mermelstein, DMD who I thank for the photographs.

What should you discuss with the dentist?

When discussing the treatment with a patient certain questions are common. One is that their friend had a lot of trouble and do I think they will have trouble? Not sure. We cannot compare. It could involve their physical health, their aftercare, and the difficulty or ease they had taking medications and following instructions.

The other question is, "My dentist took x-rays, so why do you have to take them again?" The answer is: "Because we need three-dimensional pictures. It is becoming the "standard of care." In fact, when I discuss this with dentists, I usually advise them to have the 3D imaging done before they place implants. If they don't, and there is a problem it could be harder to explain and to handle.

Another question is, "Is there a chance my body will reject the implants?" When there is a problem, it is not really rejection. It is the failure of the bone to seal against the implant. What causes it? Bacteria in the mouth can cause it. Resistant germs can cause it. That's why most of the time we prescribe antibiotics and antiseptic mouth rinses. Premature chewing can put pressure on the implant and weaken the bond of the bone to the implant.

Smoking can also be an issue. Smoking slows the blood supply to the gums which can slow the healing. Diabetes causes altered healing because of too much sugar in the blood. There are also rare incidences of medications for osteoporosis affecting bone healing.[13]

The healing process requires bones cells to take away some less healthy bone and to deposit new healthy bone. What seems to happen with the medications, called bisphosphonates, is that they change that balance. More bone gets deposited then the body takes away. The new bone is denser with fewer blood vessels. As a result, the new bone may not have enough blood supply. Bone without blood supply is like stone or marble, and it is not healthy and can sometimes die.

If the implants are not successful what happens?

Generally speaking, the dentist can replace the implant at least once into the same site or a different site, depending on the reason you needed the implants. If the implant is to replace a single tooth, then it has to go in the same site. Therefore, the site usually needs healing time before replacing the implant. Sometimes we even need to place a bone graft to fill in the socket before replacing the implant. If it is to support a denture or multiple teeth, then you don't always need to wait because the dentist may insert the implant into a different spot.

What is the best approach?

The most important thing to remember is you need to have frank discussions with your dentist about any concerns you may have. Another thing is that second opinions are good. Any dentist that is not open to that may not be the dentist for you. Anybody who has faith in their abilities and ideas should be ready to explain their rationale. They should be willing to discuss the plan with the patient or another practitioner.

Another thing to remember is often, but not always, you get what you pay for. Not all dental materials are the same. For instance, if you have a cap that is porcelain and metal, that metal can be 40% to 60% gold. We call this high noble metal. It can be metal that has 25% gold called noble metal. It could have less than 25% gold called nonprecious metal.[14]

Those three metals may respond to the porcelain the same way, but the cost is going to be different because the value of the metals is different. So if you are getting a second opinion, you need to ask about the quality of the materials.

In our office, we only use the highest quality materials. We use major brand implants, and there are a lot of different ones. There are many that are good. I won't to mention them all because I'm sure to leave some out, but there are also "clones". Some practitioners' follow rules that the FDA has in which they produce something that looks like the original implant and therefore should function like it. Sometimes they do and sometimes they don't. So you have to make sure you know what you are getting and what you are paying for.

SECTION III

What are the Critical Issues?

Dentists need to stay continually informed of new research and trends in the field of dentistry to provide their patients with the best care. Their professional learning occurs through multiple opportunities for collaboration, membership in professional organizations, and updates in professional journals.

Critical issues focus on new diagnoses and infection identification, improved treatments, and cultural impacts of dentistry within the community. Dentistry serves the individual and the public as specialists and advocates. The community relies on their medical expertise. By continuing to remain updated on current trends, dentists not only provide interventions but preventions for future health needs.

Chapter 5: Current Trends in Dentistry

Chapter 5: **Current Trends in Dentistry**

What is P. Gingivalis?

In November of 2015,[15] the Journal of Infection and Immunology published a study and it discussed the activity of a particular bacteria called porphyromonas gingivalis, also known as p. gingivalis. It is a common germ or bacteria that causes periodontitis. They discovered that the same germ, p. gingivalis that causes periodontitis also boosts enzymes that cause inflammation in the smooth muscles in the walls of arteries. The first author Boxi Zhang, a Ph.D. student, stated that the research clarifies the mechanism the timely association of periodontitis and cardiovascular disease. Our aim now is to find biomarkers that can help us diagnose and treat both diseases.

Are there cultural factors leading to periodontitis?

Previously we mentioned local aggressive periodontitis, but what we didn't discuss is that it affects 2% of African American children. There is an oral biologist at the Rutgers Dental School in Newark, New Jersey that's tracked more than 2,500 Newark children since 2007 to chart the progression of what they describe as a rare form of gum disease that afflicts African American children.[16]

The disease, which is called localized aggressive periodontitis has a genetic basis and affects 2% of children ages 11-17. They received a grant from the National Institute of Health to pinpoint biological markers in saliva that can predict whether the bone loss will occur from the disease and which teeth it will effect before there are symptoms. Because the illness mostly affects primary incisors and molars, it can result in disfigurement and difficulty eating.

Dr. Daniel Finer stated, "If we focus on these children, it gives us an opportunity to dissect the factors that lead to bone loss and help save their teeth.[17]

Does water fluoridation impact oral hygiene?

In a video posted by the office Surgeon General on YouTube, Dr. Vivic Mertha credited water fluoridation with contributing to a dramatic decline in the prevalence and severity of tooth decay.[18] Community water fluoridation helps us meet these goals and as it is one of the most cost-efficient and equitable and safe measures communities can take to prevent tooth decay and improve oral health. He praised advocates and community leaders for their effort in fighting to make water fluoridation a reality in all communities across the country. The problem is it doesn't exist in certain places. So people ask, "Why isn't the water fluoridated?"

There is a list ranking states using water fluoridation, and state of New Jersey is at the bottom of that list. Because New Jersey is a home rule state, which means, unless every community consents, there will never be 100% water fluoridation in New Jersey. Another reason is there are a lot of people that object putting fluoride in water. But today 75% of the population in the United States is served by public water utilities and receives the benefit of optimally fluoride water. Studies show community water fluoridation prevents at least 25% of tooth decay in children and adults even with the widespread availability from other sources.[19]

Fortunately, there are other ways to get fluoride and to prevent tooth decay, such as fluoride in vitamins and toothpaste. It was the surgeon general that said, "We know so much of our health is determined by zip code rather than genetic code" [20] That is why creating a culture of disease prevention by community efforts, and ensuring health equity for all is one of our highest priorities.

How do dentists stay on top of current trends?

There is value in maintaining membership in the local dental society and the American Dental Association. Many people just assume that all dentists are members. Well, that is not true. In the United States, membership in the American Dental Association is described as a tripartite membership. It means that you belong to your local dental society, which in my case is the Essex County NJ Dental Society (ECDS). You belong to the state dental association which in my case is the New Jersey Dental Association (NJDA), and you belong to the American Dental Association (ADA).

What is the value of the American Dental Association?

Many believe that the ADA is self-serving. That is far from the truth. The ADA serves the public and it also helps dentists who aren't members. It serves the public through scientific research, through continuing education for dentists, including what is called evidence-based dentistry, and also with publications that keep dentists aware of new trends and new techniques in dentistry.

Continuing education courses allow dentist to keep current with new advances that help their patients. The ADA and its component state societies also perform "missions of mercy" where dentist provide free care to needy patients. One such program is Give Kids a Smile that provides care for the underserved children in our communities.

What are the specialties of dentistry?

The American Dental Association recognizes nine dental specialties: Periodontics, Oral and Maxillofacial Surgery, Endodontics, Oral Pathology, Dental Public Health, Oral and Maxillofacial Radiology, Orthodontics and Dentofacial Orthopedics, Pediatric Dentistry, and Prosthodontics.[21]

Dental Public Health is the science and art of preventing and controlling dental disease and promoting community oral health by the efforts such as water fluoridation. The public serves as the patient rather than an individual.

Another specialty is Endodontics. It is the branch of dentistry concerned with what is described as the morphology, physiology, and pathology of the human dental pulp. To be an Endodontist means to be a root canal specialist.

Oral and Maxillofacial Pathology is a particular specialty that deals with the nature, identification, and management of diseases affecting the oral maxilla facial region. It investigates the problems, causes and effects of a disease. Often the diagnosis is done through microscopic examination of tissues under a microscope.

The concern of an Oral and Maxillofacial Radiology specialist focuses on the production and interpretation of images and data. Essentially, the practitioner uses x-rays to diagnose and manages diseases and conditions of the oral and maxillofacial region.

The next specialty is Oral and Maxillofacial Surgery which includes the diagnosis and treatment of illness, injuries, and defects involving both the functional and aesthetics aspects of the hard and soft tissues of the mouth. They are commonly called Oral Surgeons.

Orthodontics is the specialty that diagnoses, provides prevention, interception, and correction of malocclusions; as well as neuromuscular and skeletal abnormalities of the developing or mature face.

Pediatric Dentistry is the specialty that provides primary, comprehensive, and therapeutic care for infants and children right through adolescence including those with special needs.

Prosthodontics is the dental specialty pertaining to the diagnosis, treatment planning, rehabilitation, and maintenance of oral functions. It also addresses the comfort, appearance, and health associated with missing or damaged teeth.

Finally, Periodontics is that specialty of dentistry which encompasses the prevention diagnosis and treatment of diseases and the surrounding and supporting tissues of the teeth or their substitutes. This includes dental implants. Periodontists also help patients maintain the health of the function and aesthetics of their gums and teeth.

Conclusion

So to review, there are several types of gum disease. The most common type, and the one that you hear advertised on TV, is called Gingivitis. It causes the edge of the gum around the tooth to become inflamed due to bacterial plaque building up around the tooth. Usually, with proper professional cleaning followed by appropriate home care, gingivitis is reversible. Factors that might promote gingivitis are diabetes, smoking, a genetic predisposition, stress, puberty, hormonal fluctuations, pregnancy, substance abuse, HIV and certain medications. If left untreated, gingivitis can advance to periodontitis.

It is obvious that this book cannot discover every dental procedure available. Discussing other areas of dentistry may be a reason for another book. I primarily attempted to discuss issues that many adults encounter, but may want to learn more about. At the same time, they are the areas of dentistry that I am most adept at and have dedicated my career mastering.

The most important take away for you is that you should ask questions. What are my options? What are the expected results? How long will it take? What will it cost? How long will it last? What are that possible pitfalls or complications? Will you teach me how to maintain my dental health?

These are my final words. I encourage you to visit your dentist regularly for cleanings, checkups and any needed care. Putting off necessary treatment can only allow a problem to worsen.

Do your home care! Preventive care is the most cost effective treatment. If you, dear reader, would like additional information about any dental issues, feel free to contact me. It would be my pleasure to answer any questions that you may have. And thank you very much for your interest in my life's work.

Dr. Gregory LaMorte

lamortedds@gmail.com

http://www.drlamorte.com/

Healthy Smile, Happy Body!

Citations

1. Dr. Thomas Fuller ((1654 - 1734), Gnomologia, 1732
    http://www.quotationspage.com/search.php3?homesearch=heal
    th&page=3
2. http://www.mouthhealthy.org/en/adults-under-40/concerns
3. http://www.mouthhealthy.org/en/pregnancy/
4. http://www.cdc.gov/OralHealth/periodontal_disease/index.htm
5. https://www.perio.org/consumer/pregnancy-treatment
6. https://www.perio.org/consumer/men and
    https://www.perio.org/consumer/women.htm
7. Journal of Periodontology. 2010 Jun; 81(6):864-9. Association
    between periodontal disease and prostate-specific antigen levels
    in chronic prostatitis patients. Joshi N1, Bissada NF, Bodner D,
    Maclennan GT, Narendran S, Jurevic R, Skillicorn R.
8. American Heart Journal The prevalence and incidence of coronary
    heart disease is significantly increased in periodontitis: A meta-
    analysis Amol Ashok Bahekar, MD Sarabjeet Singh, MD Sandeep
    Saha, MD Janos Molnar, MD Rohit Arora, MD, Department of
    Cardiology, Chicago Medical School - North Chicago Veterans
    Affairs Medical Center, Chicago, IL
9. Ibid
10. Journal of Dental Research, October 2012 91: 914-920 Prevalence
    of Periodontitis in Adults in the United States: 2009 and 2010 P.I.
    Eke B.A. Dye L. Wei G.O. Thornton-Evans
    R.J. Genco4 on behalf of the participating members of the CDC
    Periodontal Disease Surveillance workgroup: James Beck
    (University of North Carolina, Chapel Hill, USA), Gordon Douglass
    (Past President, American Academy of Periodontology), Roy Page
    (University of Washington, Seattle, USA), Gary Slade (University
    of North Carolina, Chapel Hill, USA), George W. Taylor (University
    of Michigan, Ann Arbor, USA), Wenche Borgnakke (University of
    Michigan, Ann Arbor, USA), and representatives of the American
    Academy of Periodontology

11. Journal of Clinical Dentistry 2015;26:109–114)
    Case Series Report of 66 Refractory Maintenance Patients
    Evaluating the Effectiveness of Topical Oxidizing Agents
12. R. Bruce Cochrane, DDS, MS IA Periodontics and Prosthodontics
    Fort Dodge, IA, USA Betty Sindelar, PhD, PT Ohio University
    School of Rehabilitation and Communication Sciences Athens,
    OH, USA
13. Journal of Oral Implantology Released: 6-Nov-2012 11:15 AM EST
    Success of Dental Implants Depends on Both Patient and Surgeon
14. Implant Dentistry: February 2010 - Volume 19 - Issue 1 - pp 57-64
    Smoking, Diabetes Mellitus, Periodontitis, and Supportive
    Periodontal Treatment as Factors Associated With Dental Implant
    Survival: A Long-Term Retrospective Evaluation of Patients
    Followed for Up to 10 Years
    Anner, Rachel DMD; Grossmann, Yoav DMD; Anner, Yael; Levin,
    Liran DMD
15. http://www.ada.org/en/member-center/oral-health-
    topics/dental-materials
16. Gingipains from the Periodontal Pathogen Porphyromonas
    gingivalis Play a Significant Role in Regulation of Angiopoietin 1
    and Angiopoietin 2 in Human Aortic Smooth Muscle Cells.
    Infect. Immun.
    Infect Immun 2015 Nov 17; 83(11):4256-65. Epub 2015 Aug 17.
    Boxi Zhang, Hazem Khalaf, Allan Sirsjö, Torbjörn Bengtsson
17. Rare Gum Disease Among African-American Children is Focus of
    Rutgers Study
    Rutgers Today Wednesday, February 18, 2015, By Carrie Stetler
18. ibid
19. https://www.youtube.com/watch?v=VPEu00-gW2I&noredirect=1
20. Achievements in Public Health, 1900-1999: Fluoridation of
    Drinking Water to Prevent Dental Caries CDC MMWR Weekly
    October 22, 1999 /48(41); 933-940
21. https://www.youtube.com/watch?list=PL050E3432C9D6BE2B&v=
    VPEu00-gW2I http://www.ada.org/en/education-careers/careers-
    in-dentistry/dental-specialties/specialty-definitions

Glossary

Acetaminophen: A non-aspirin pain reliever that you can buy without a prescription. An overdose can cause irreversible liver damage. Be careful to take as directed.

Acute: A problem that comes on suddenly.

Adult-onset diabetes: A health condition that develops in adults, in which they are unable to control the level of sugar in the blood.

Antibiotic prophylaxis: The use of antibiotics before treatment to prevent an infection. Also called premedication.

Anticoagulants: Medications used to keep blood clots from forming in the body, also known as blood thinners.

Bacterial endocarditis: A serious, but rare, infection involving the heart lining.

Bisphosphonate: A medicine that treats osteopenia or osteoporosis. In rare cases, it causes jaw bone problems.

Bleaching: The process of lightening the teeth to remove stains. The process usually involves some type of peroxide.

Bone augmentation: Building up the bone around a tooth, dental implants, or sinuses.

Biopsy: The process of removing tissue for microscopic evaluation and disease diagnosis by a pathologist.

Bone loss: A decrease in the amount of bone that supports a tooth or implant.

Buccal: Referring to the tooth surface that faces toward the cheeks or lips.

Caries: The dental term for tooth decay.

Cavity: A hole in a tooth due to decay.

Clinical trial: Research studies of the preventative or therapeutic effectiveness and/or safety of a treatment or medicine.

Codeine: A prescription pain reliever usually combined in a pill with acetaminophen or aspirin. It is known for side effects, including sleepiness, dizziness, constipation, and physical dependence.

Cosmetic dentistry: Any services provided by a dentist solely for the purpose of improving your appearance, not your health.

Crown: 1.The part of the tooth covered with shiny, smooth enamel. 2. An artificial or synthetic crown is a single, artificial tooth that fits over a real tooth that has been specially shaped. It can also be designed to fit over a dental implant. Also known as a cap.

Decay: The softening of tooth structure caused by acid from bacteria.

Deciduous teeth: These are the first teeth a child gets. They are also called primary teeth, baby teeth, and sometimes milk teeth.

Dental bridge: This is a dental appliance that fills the space left by a missing tooth or teeth. It is held in place by attaching to natural teeth or implants. It can be removable or cemented (fixed) in place.

Dental erosion: Dental erosion is the thinning or wearing away of the hard enamel coating of a tooth.

Dentifrice: Another name for toothpaste.

Dentures: Artificial teeth. They can replace a whole set of teeth called a complete denture or just some teeth, called a partial denture. **Denture adhesives:** A paste or powder that can be used to hold dentures in place.

Distal: Referring to the tooth surface that faces away from the midline of the either dental arch.

Dry mouth: Also called xerostomia; a condition that results from an inadequate flow of saliva. I can be a side effect of medication or, sometimes, part of the aging process.

Enamel: The hard calcified tissue covering the surface the tooth above the gum.

Extraction: To remove a tooth.

Floss: String used to remove bacteria (plaque) between the teeth where a toothbrush does not reach. It is usually made from nylon or plastic.

Fluoride: A supplement that helps prevent tooth decay (cavities). Some communities add it to water. Some children get it vitamins. It can be applied by a dentist.

Gingiva: The dental term for gums.

Gingivitis: Inflammation of the soft gum tissue.

Ibuprofen: A medication related to aspirin that relieves pain. You can buy it without a prescription. Can cause side effects that can affect the stomach or the heart.

Implant: An artificial tooth root that dentists put into the jaw bone. The dentist can put an artificial tooth (a crown) on the implant. Sometimes, implants are used to hold bridges or dentures in place.

Incisal: Referring to the thin edge of a front tooth.

Interdental cleaner: A device used to clean between the teeth, such as floss.

Intraoral: Inside the mouth.

Jaw: A common name for either the maxilla (upper jaw) or the mandible (lower jaw.)

Lingual: Referring to the tooth surface of a lower tooth, which face toward the tongue.

Loading: The process of a dentist attaching the artificial tooth or dentures onto an implant.

Malocclusion: This term is used to describe teeth that don't line up correctly in the mouth. They may be too far apart, crooked or may not come together right when you bite down.

Mesial: Referring to the tooth surface that faces toward the midline of the dental arch.

Molars: These are the big teeth that in the back of the mouth. We use them to grind food into small bits to aid digestion.

Mouth Rinse: An oral rinse that can be used to freshen breath, help prevent or control tooth decay, reduce plaque, prevent or reduce gingivitis, reduce the formation of tartar, or a combination of these effects, usually available without a prescription.

NSAIDs: An abbreviation for nonsteroidal anti-inflammatory drugs. A group of medicines that relieve pain and inflammation.

Occlusal: Referring to the tooth surface that is the actual biting surface of a back tooth.

Opioids: Prescription medications for pain. Codeine is one type. Others are hydrocodone and oxycodone.

Oral: Pertaining to the mouth.

Oral hygiene: Activities you do to keep your mouth clean. These include brushing your teeth, cheeks, tongue and dentures. They also can include using mouthwash or dental floss, or having a dentist or hygienist clean your teeth.

Oral Lichen Planus: A type of autoimmune disease that can be seen in the mouth. It may appear as white patches; red, swollen tissues; or open sores in the mouth.

Orthodontic treatment: Orthodontic treatment is used to straighten teeth. It can be done with 'braces" or removable dental appliances.

Osteonecrosis of the Jaw: A disease signified by slow, delayed healing of the jawbone, sometimes referred to as ONJ.

Palatal: Referring to the tooth surface of an upper tooth that faces toward the roof of the mouth.

Peri-Implantitis: An infection of the gum and/or bone around an implant. It can cause bone loss.

Periodontal disease: When plaque is not removed, it can cause gums to separate and pull away from your teeth. Your gums may also become inflamed and bleed.

Periodontitis: A form of gum and bone disease in the mouth which can lead to tooth loss.

Plaque: A soft, sticky, thin layer of bacteria that forms on your teeth.

Primary Teeth: The first set of teeth that you get when you are a child. These are sometimes called baby teeth or milk teeth.

Dental Prophylaxis or a "dental prophy": The removal of plaque, calculus (tartar) and stains from the teeth, also called a prophy or teeth cleaning.

Pulp: The blood supply and nerves inside a tooth.

Quadrant: One of the four equal sections into which the dental arches can be divided. It begins at the midline of the arch and extends to the last tooth.

Radiograph: A picture of the bones or teeth inside the body. It also is called an X-ray.

Recession: When the gum line moves down a tooth exposing more of the tooth.

Root canal treatment: The removal of the soft tissues inside a tooth. The tooth is filled form tip to tip with a resin to prevent tissue from growing back into the tooth.

Sealant: A plastic coating that can be put on the tops of teeth. They help prevent cavities.

Sinuses: The air spaces in the bones of your face, located in the forehead and on either side of the nose.

Sjögren Syndrome: An illness in which the immune system attacks the body's own cells by mistake. It mainly causes dry mouth and dry eyes.

Staining: Discoloration of tooth surfaces. Can happen as the result of injury, genetics, smoking, some medications, drinking of coffee or tea but is ultimately a part of aging.

Stomatitis: An irritation of any of the soft tissues of the mouth: lips, gums, cheeks, tongue, floor or roof of the mouth.

Temporomandibular Joint disorders: These are problems in your jaw joints that can cause pain. Also called TMD.

Tooth decay: A hole in the tooth caused by the acid in plaque. The more common name is cavity.

Tooth extraction: The removal of a tooth from the bone socket and surrounding gums.

Topical: Refers to medications that are applied to the surface of the body.

Unerupted: A tooth that has not pushed through the gum.

Veneer: Thin, custom-made shells crafted of tooth-colored materials designed to cover the front surfaces of teeth.

Wisdom teeth: The last teeth to come in during young adulthood, also called third molars.

Xerostomia: Decreased salivary secretion that produces a dry and sometimes burning sensation. Also called dry mouth.

X-ray: See radiograph.

Zygomatic bone or zygoma: Bone on either side of the face that forms the cheek prominence.